The Wonderful Book of
KITTENS

Dedicated to my wife for
allowing me the time to
create and play.

Also dedicated to everyone
that suffers in their golden years.
May you find some joy
in this book.

Books in this series:

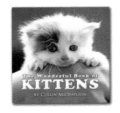 KITTENS

PUPPIES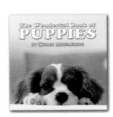

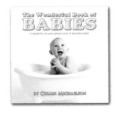 BABIES

BIRDS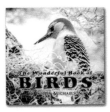

The Wonderful Book of
KITTENS

BY COLLIN MICHAELSON

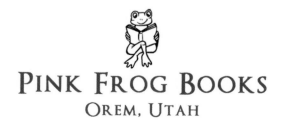

PINK FROG BOOKS

OREM, UTAH

The Wonderful Book of
KITTENS

ISBN: 9798645959647

First Printing, 2020.

Published by Pink Frog Books
www.PinkFrogBooks.com

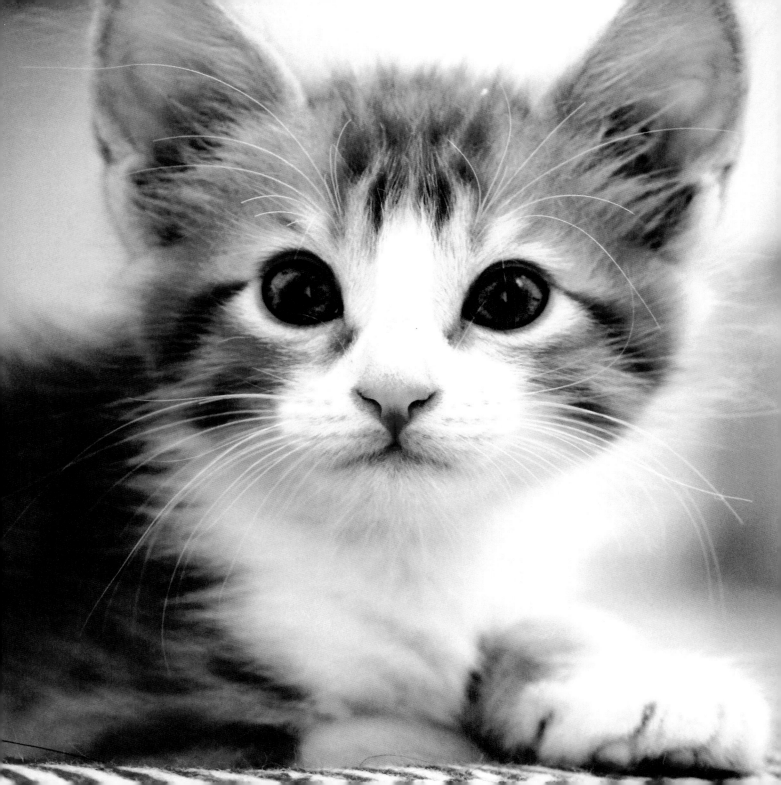

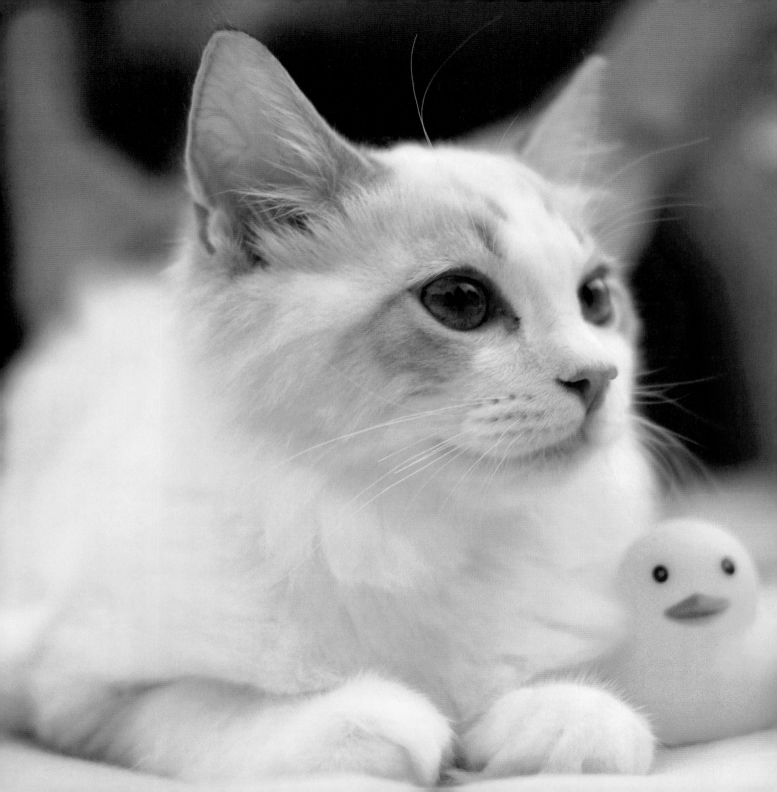

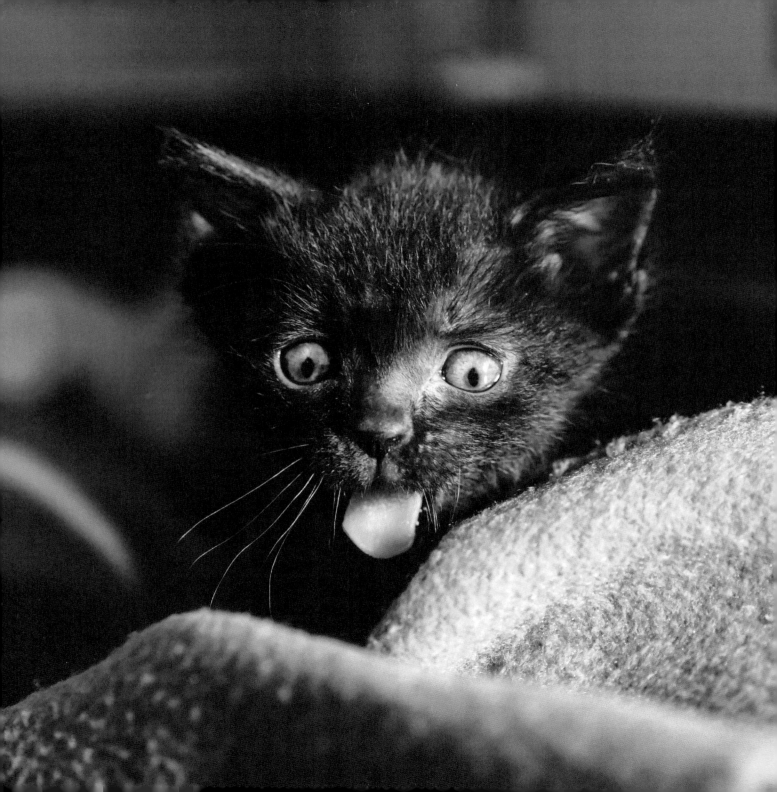

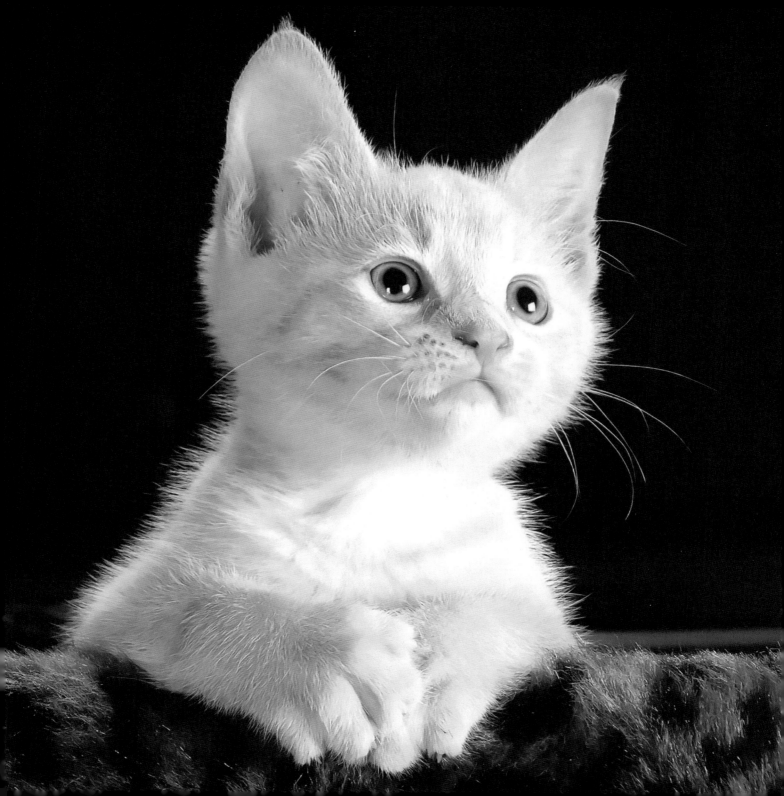

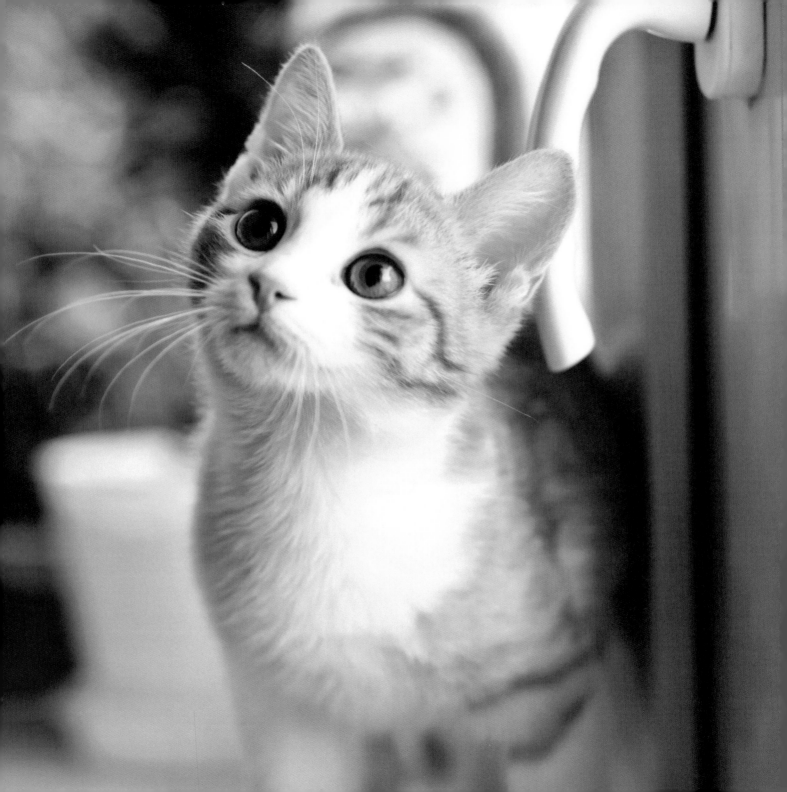

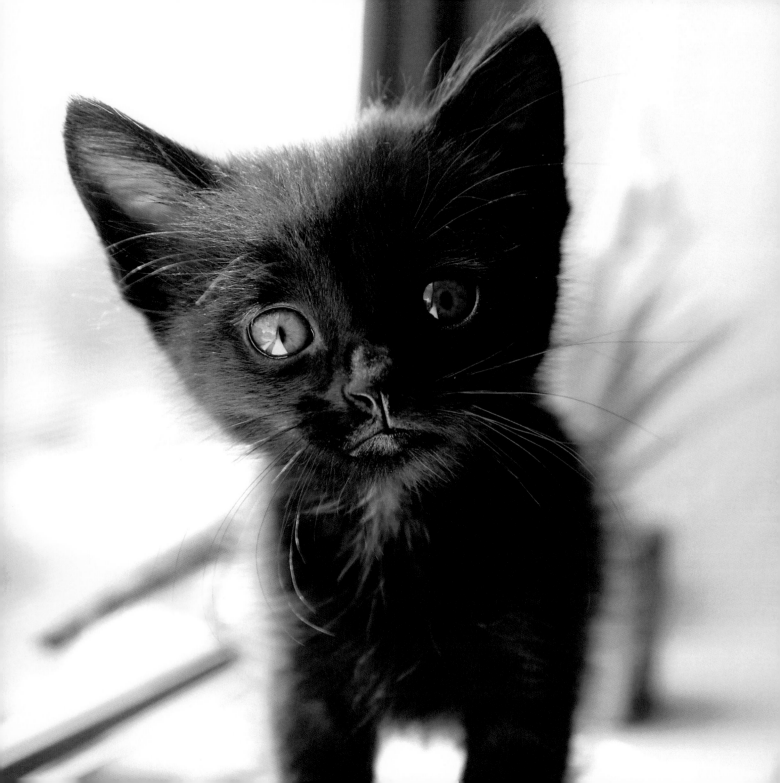

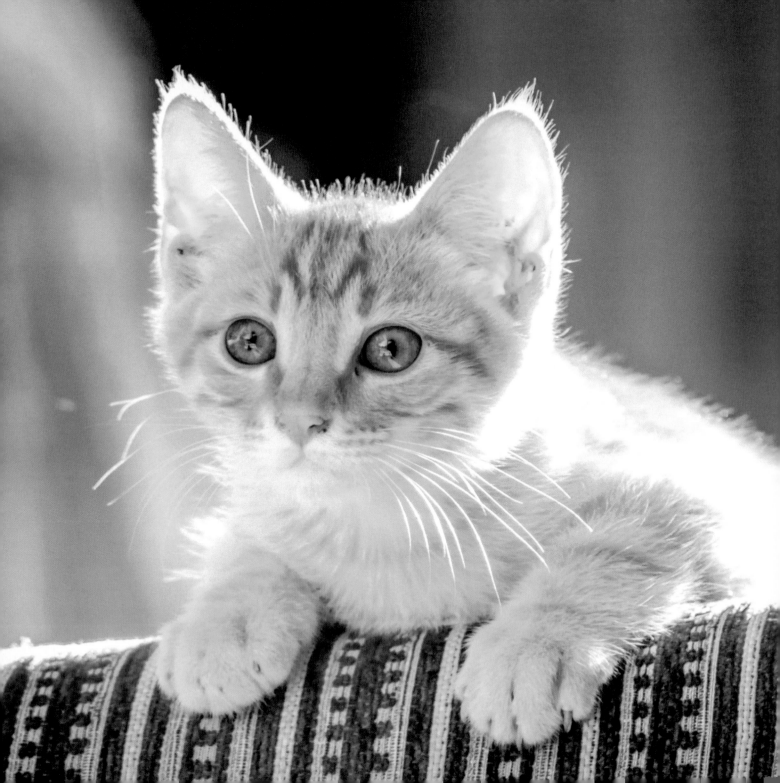

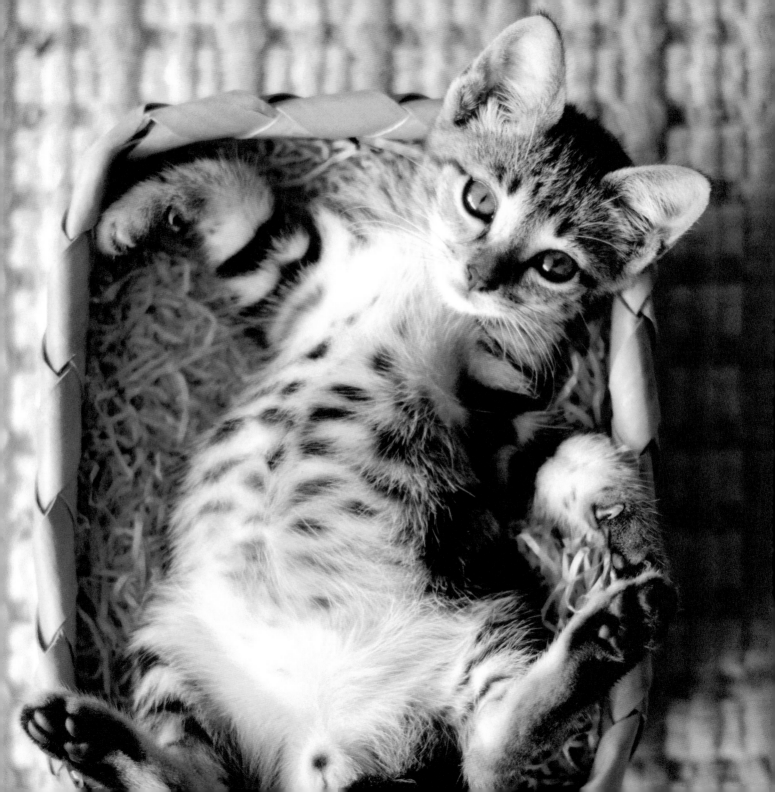

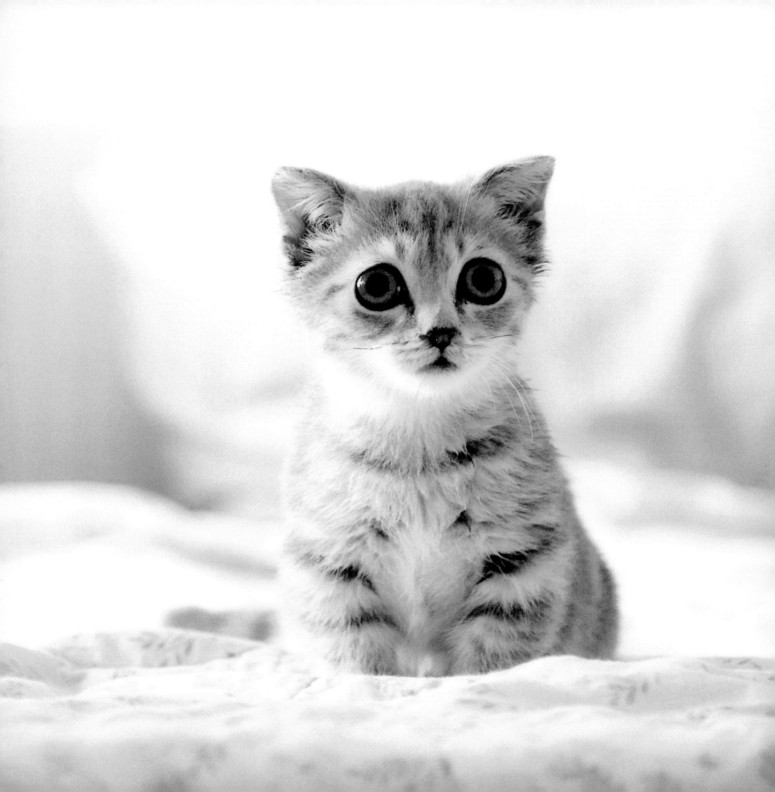

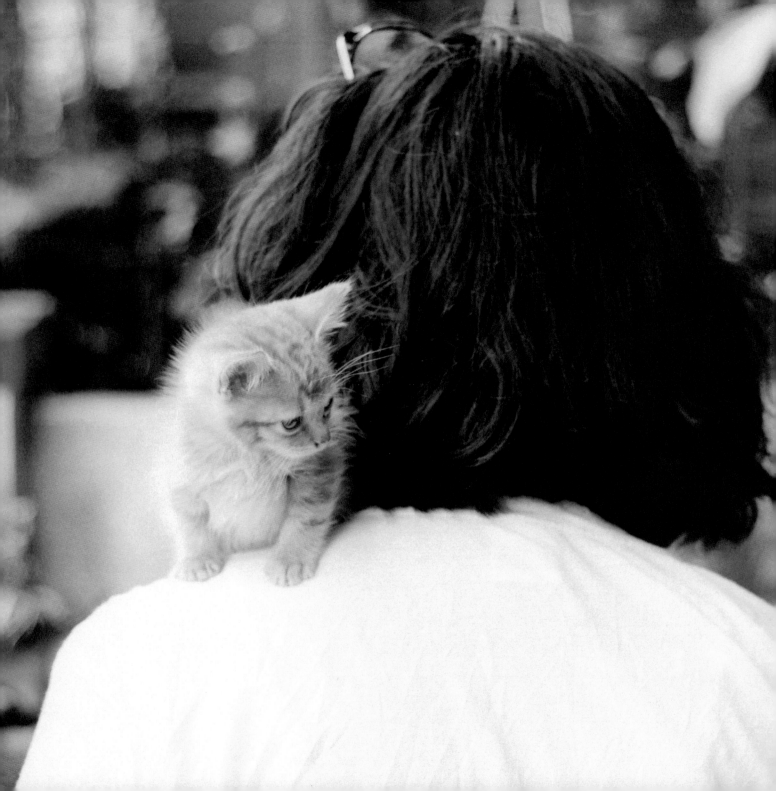

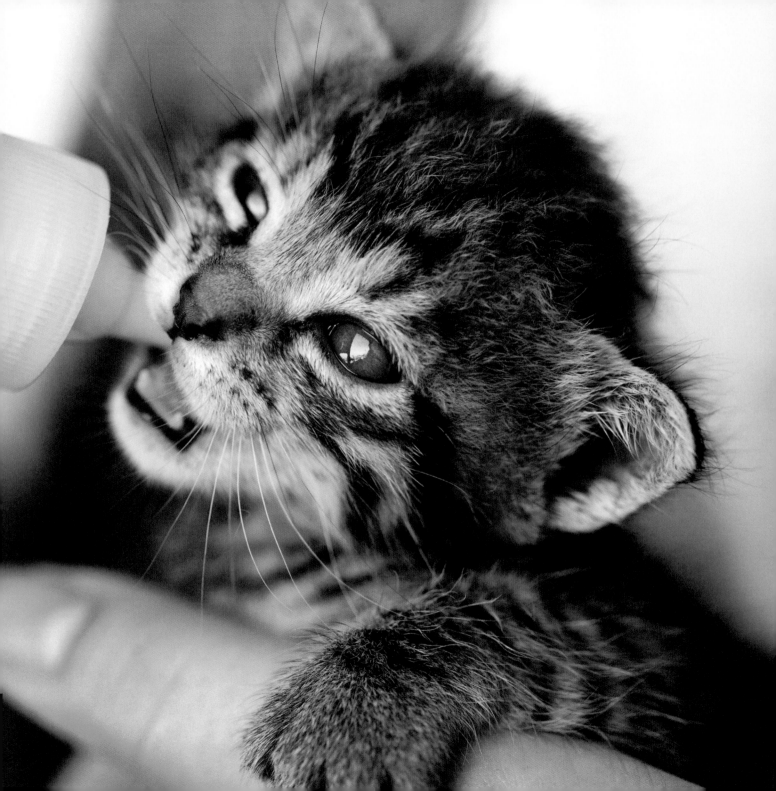

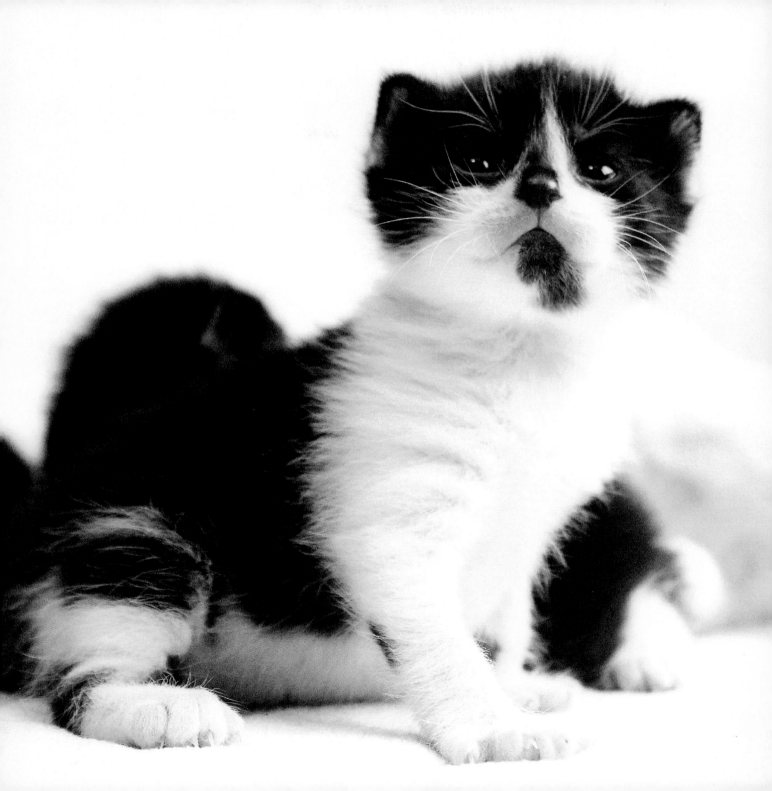

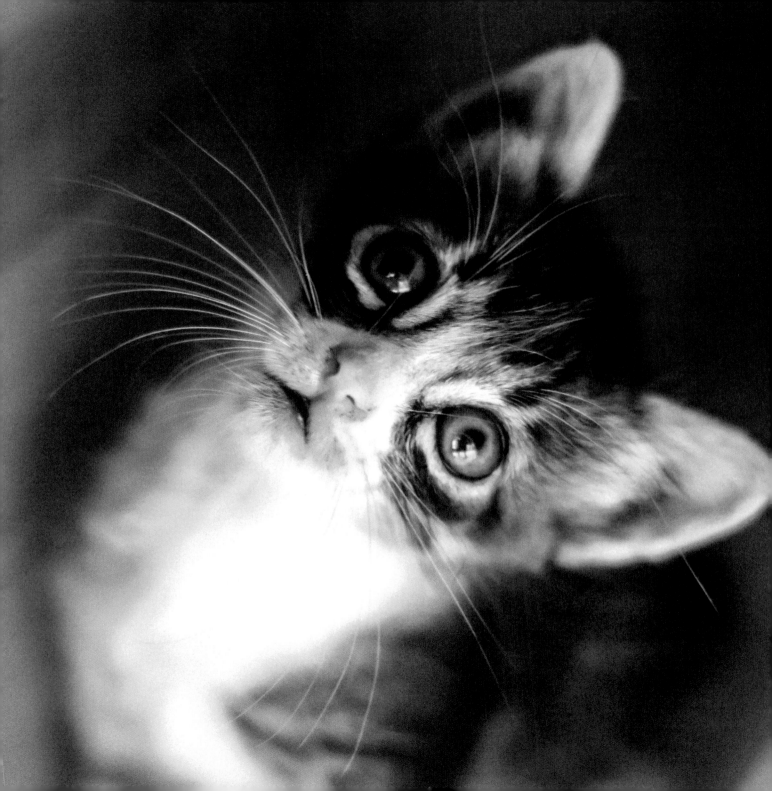

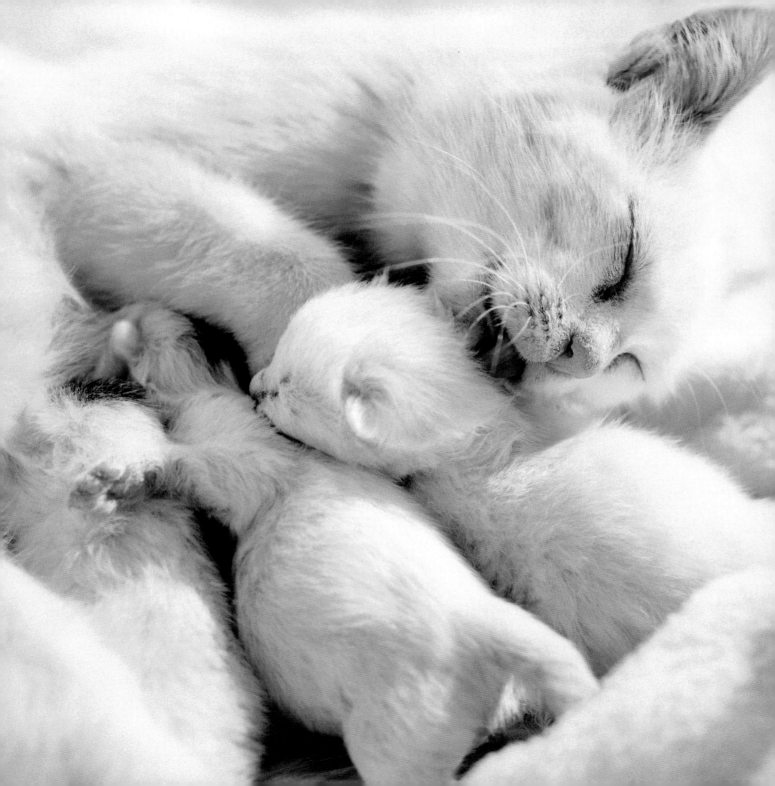

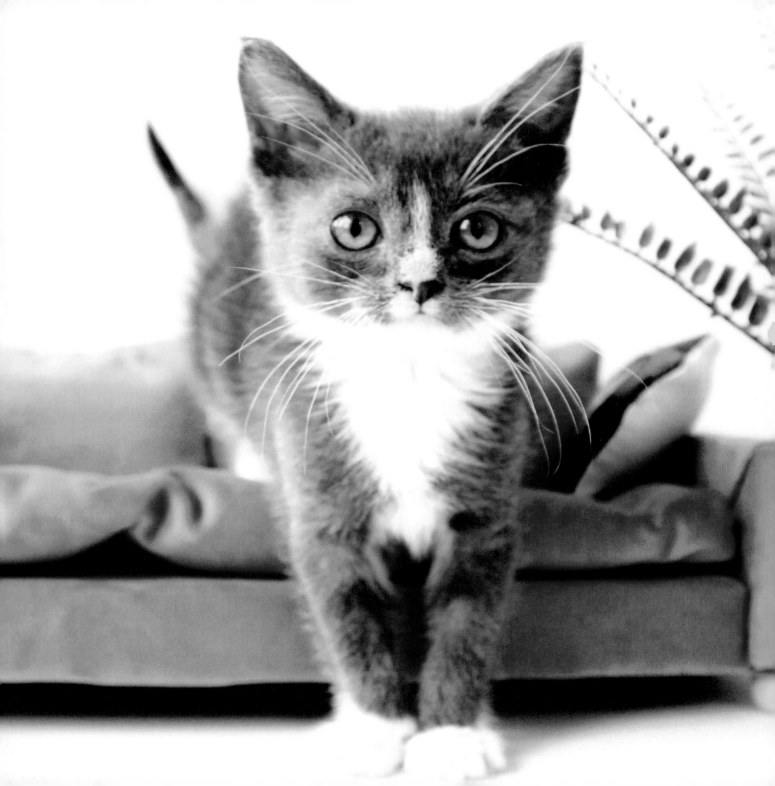

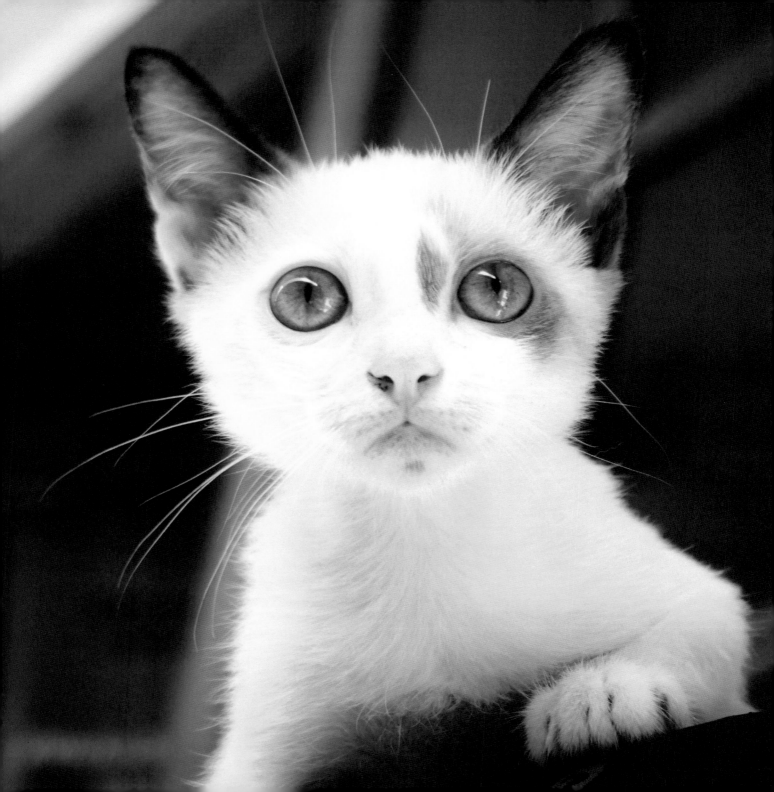

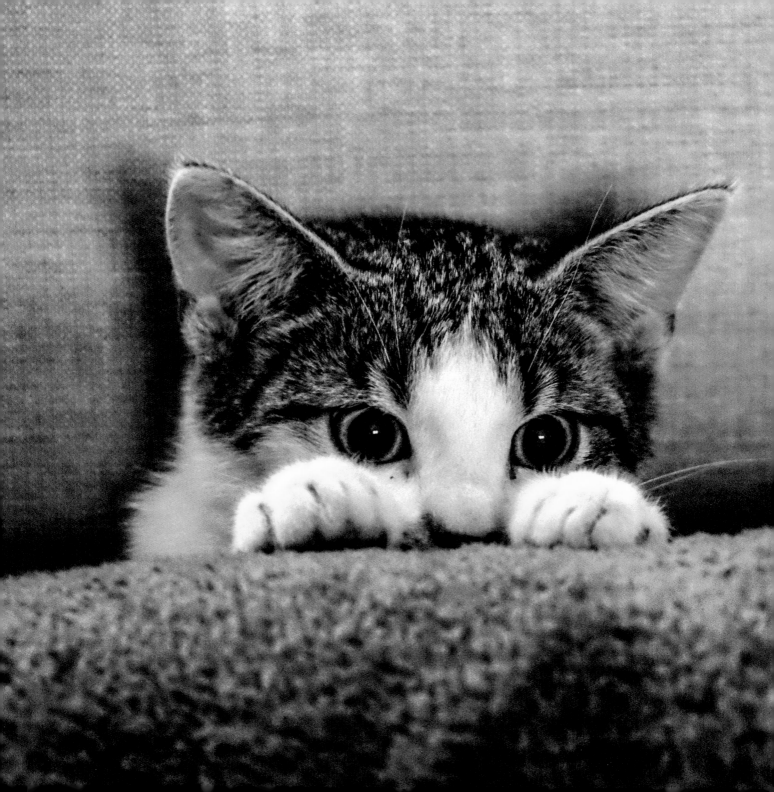

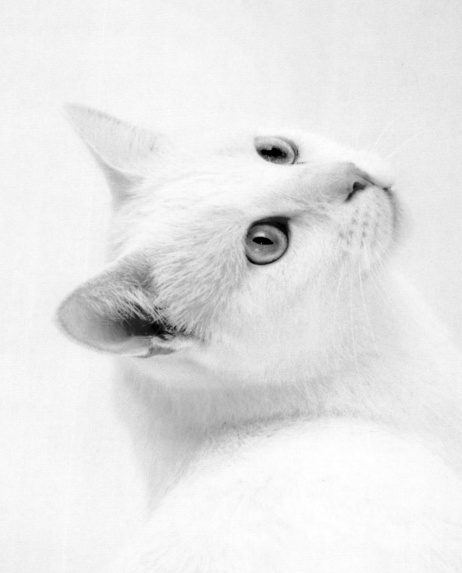

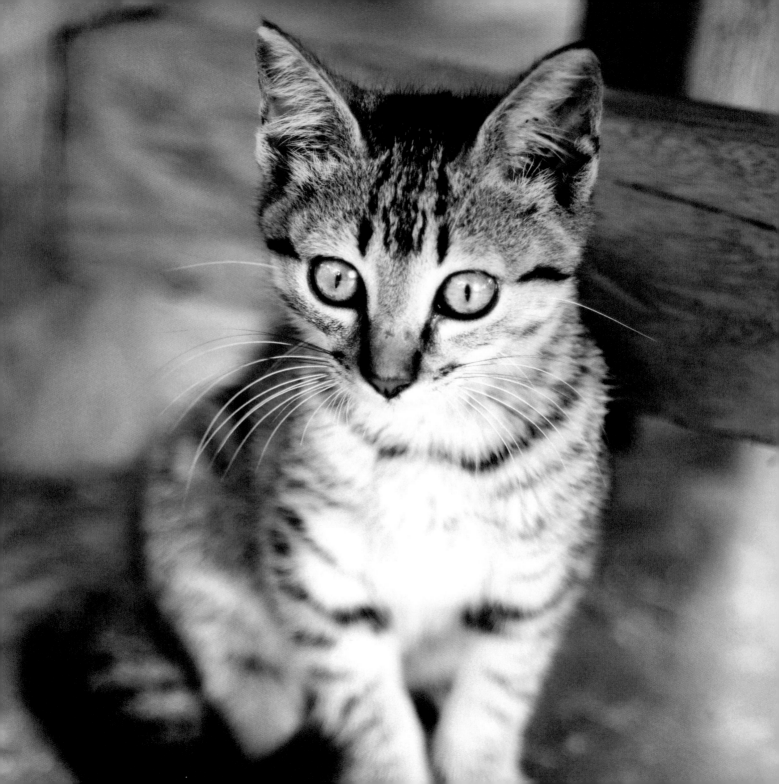

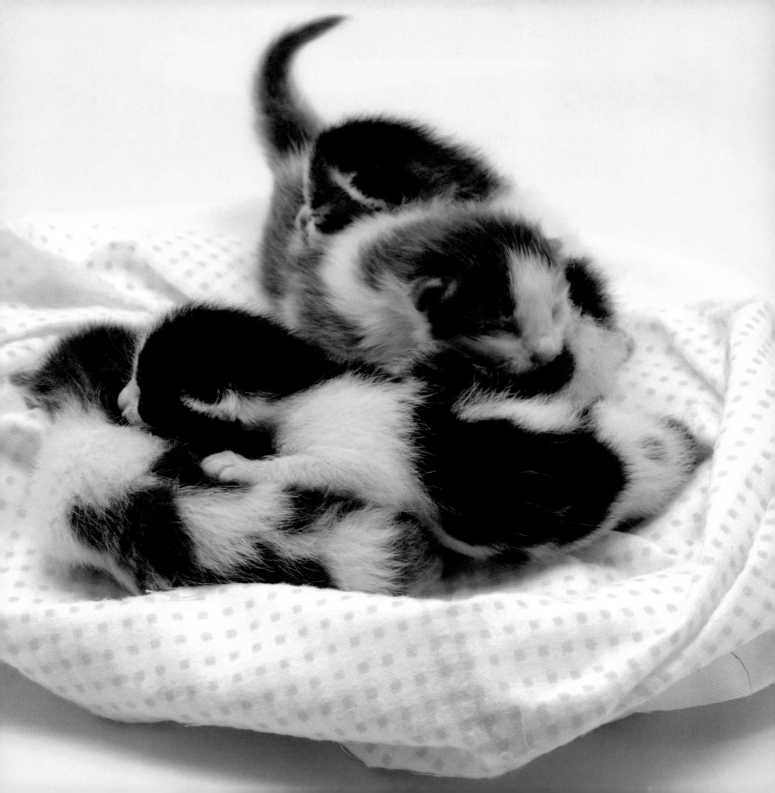

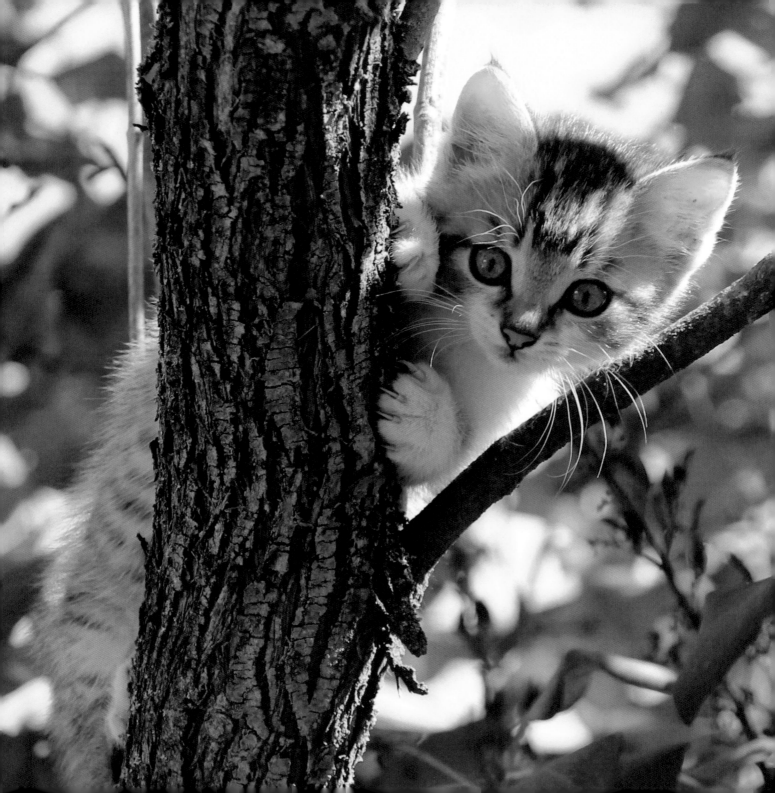

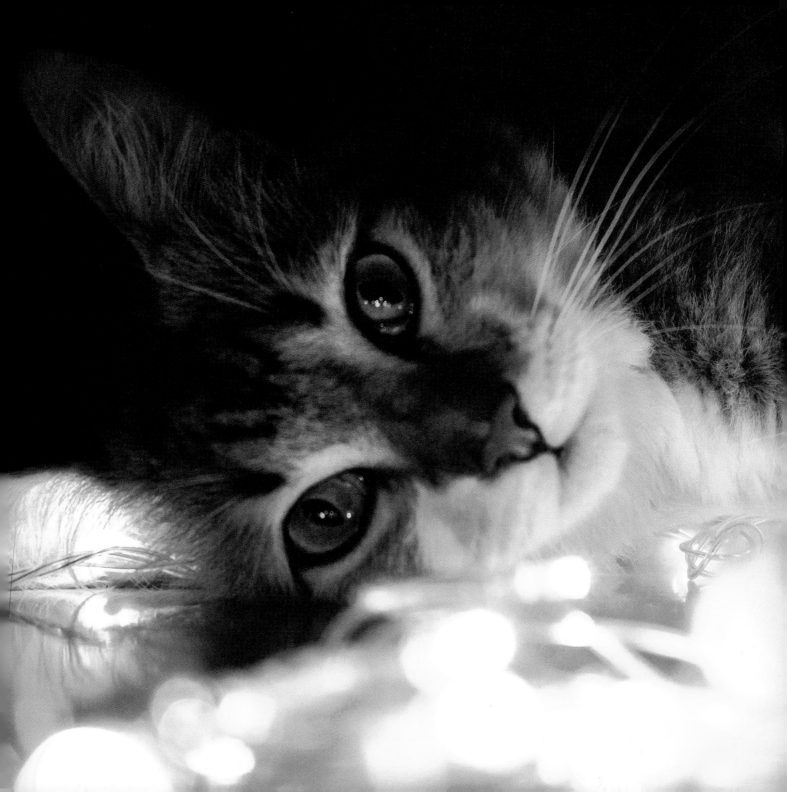

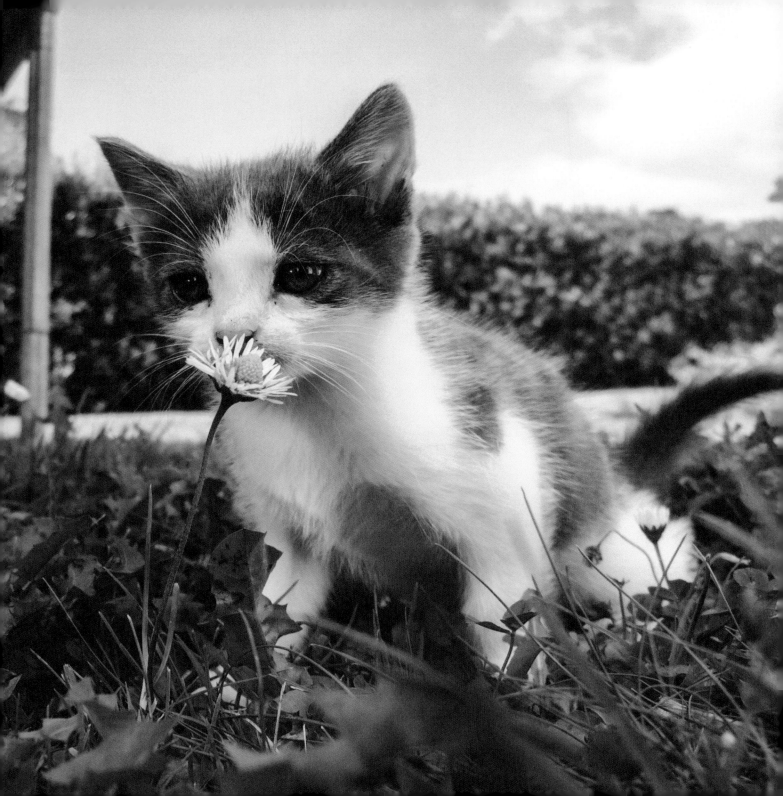

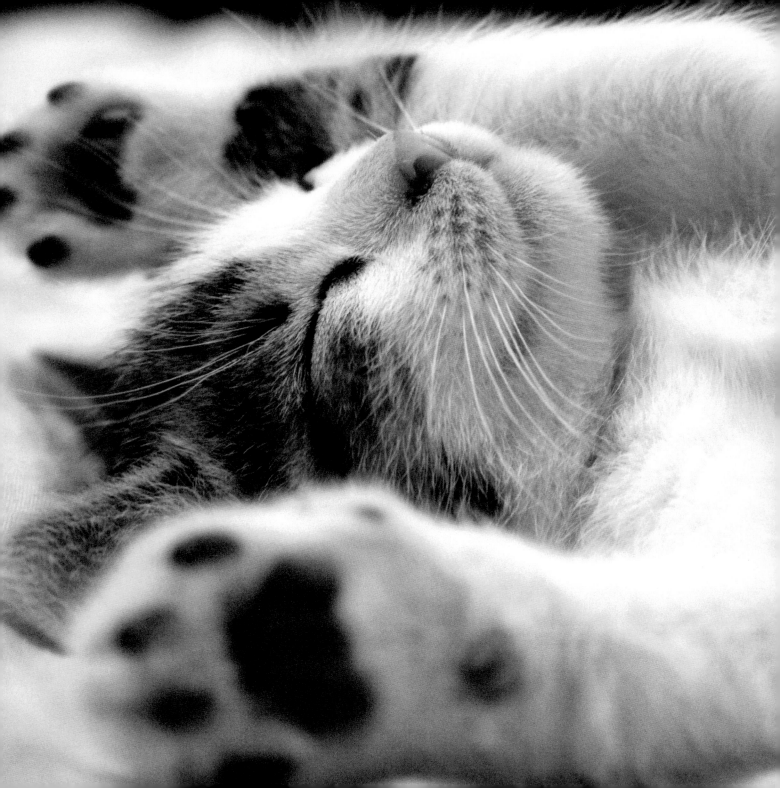

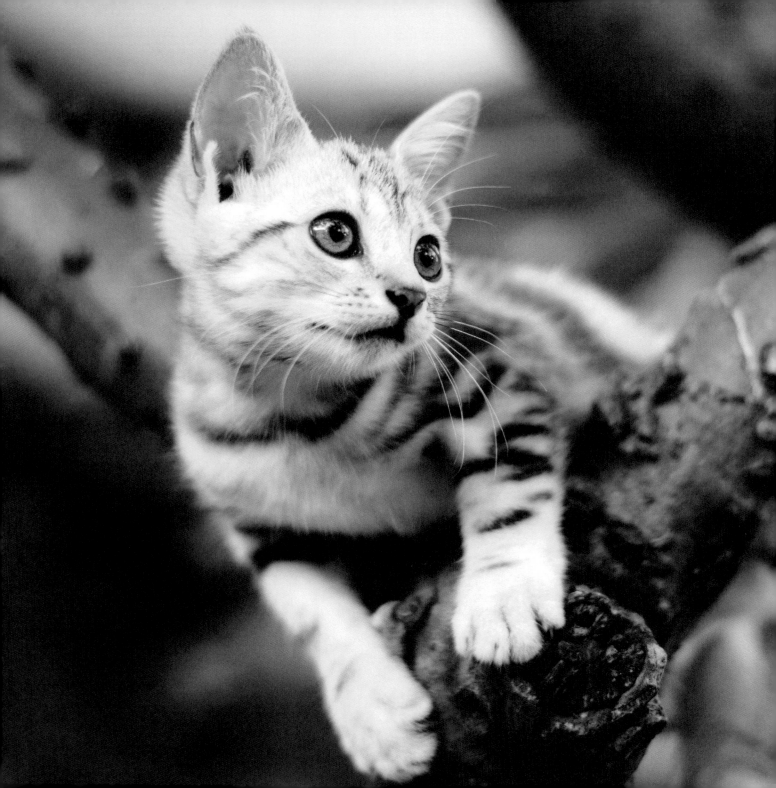

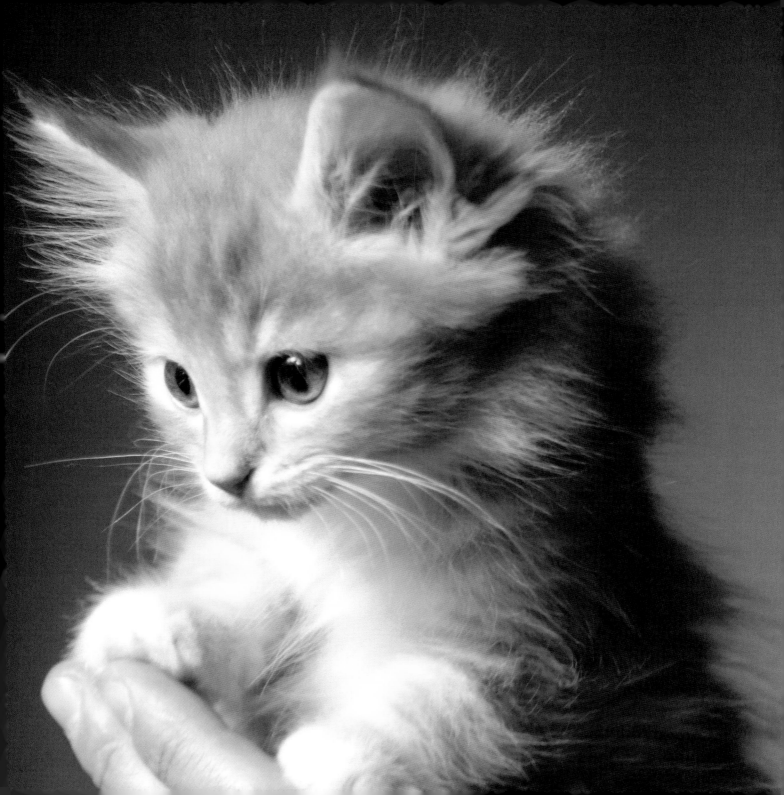

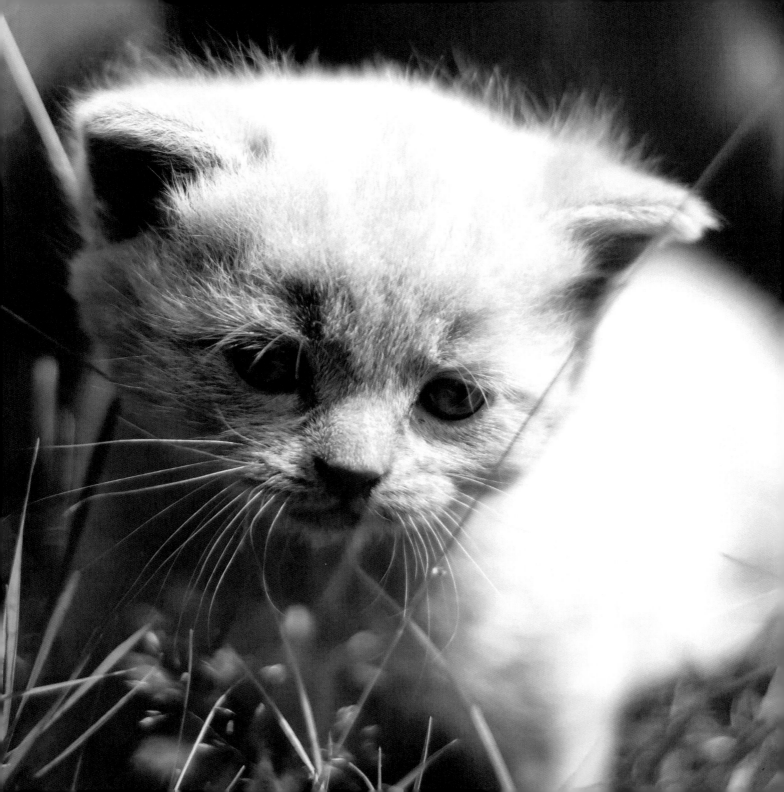

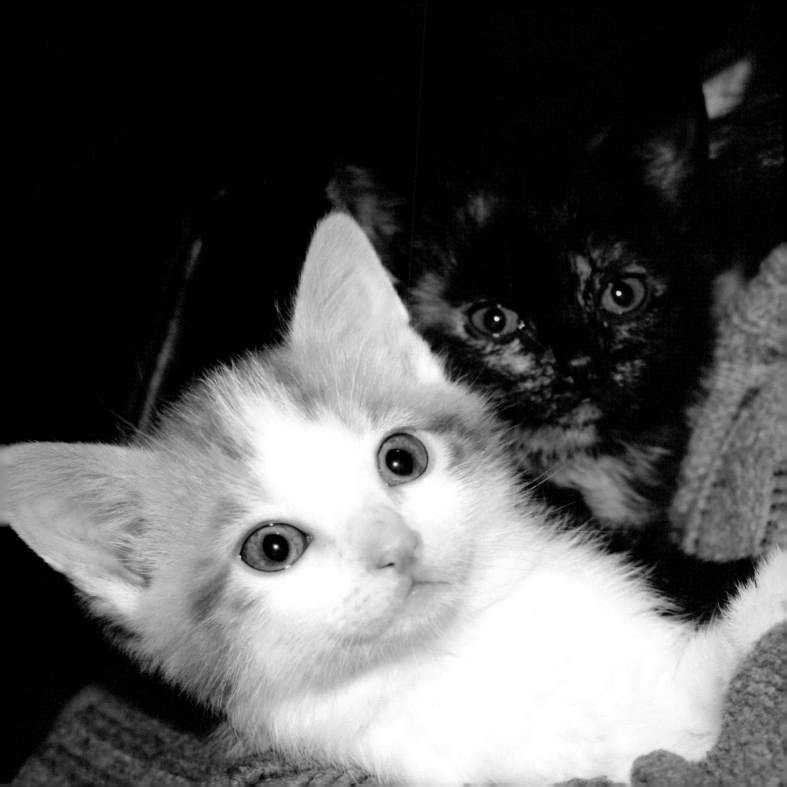

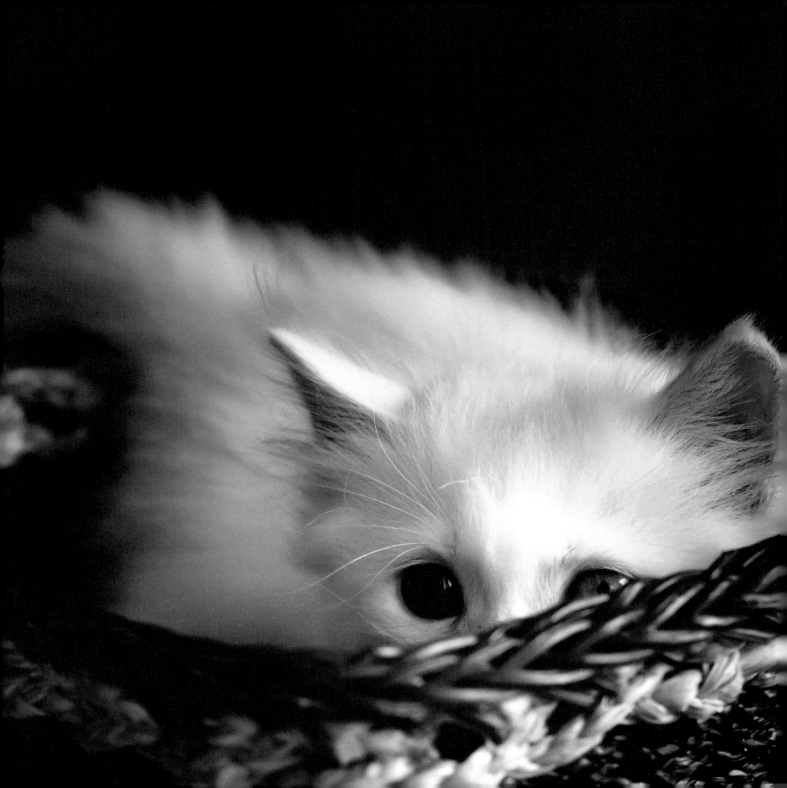

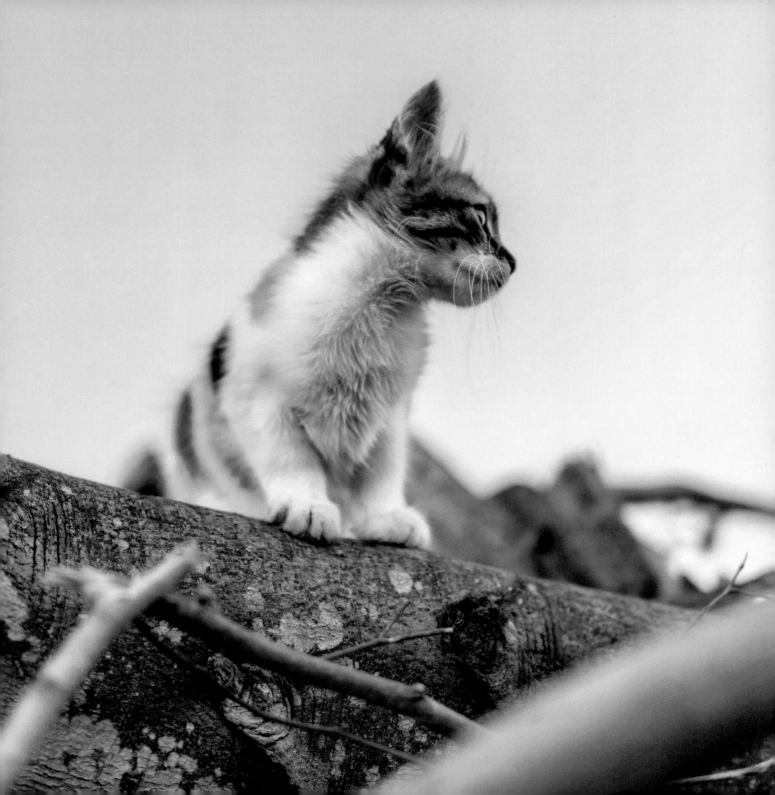

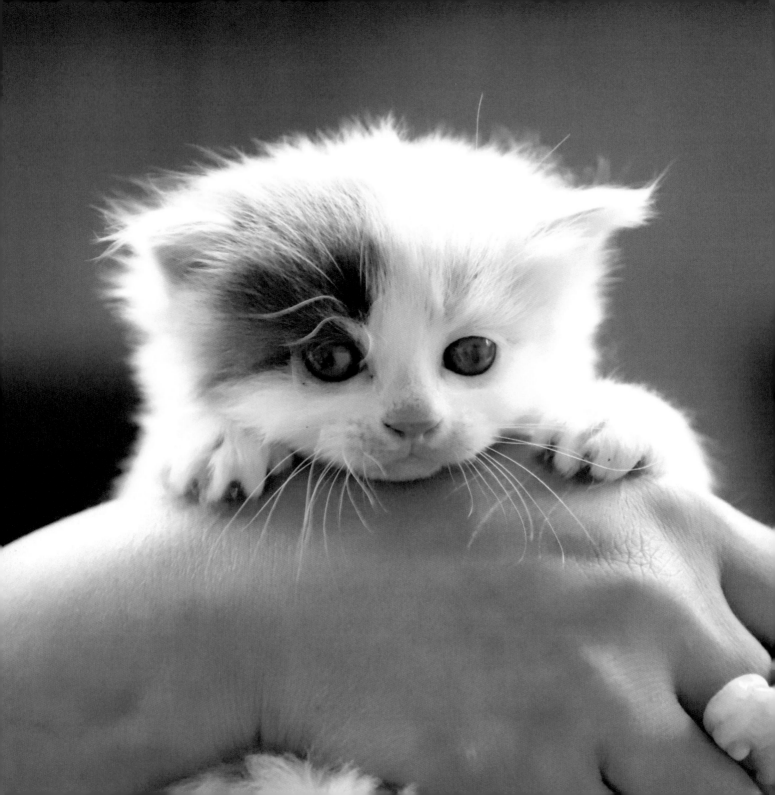

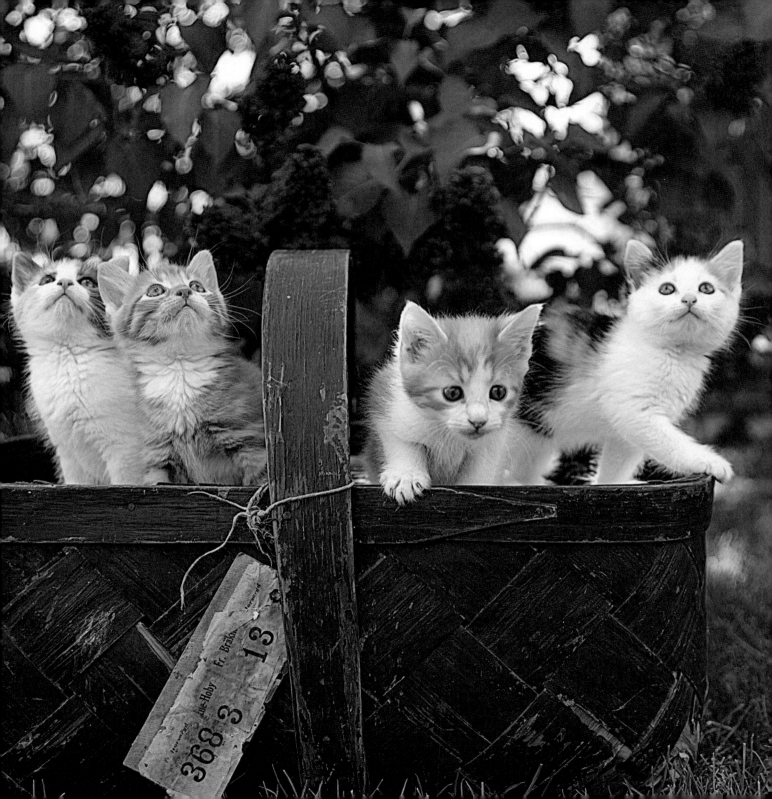

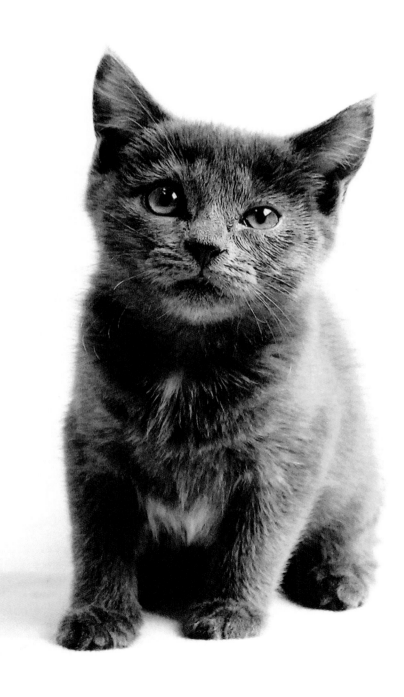

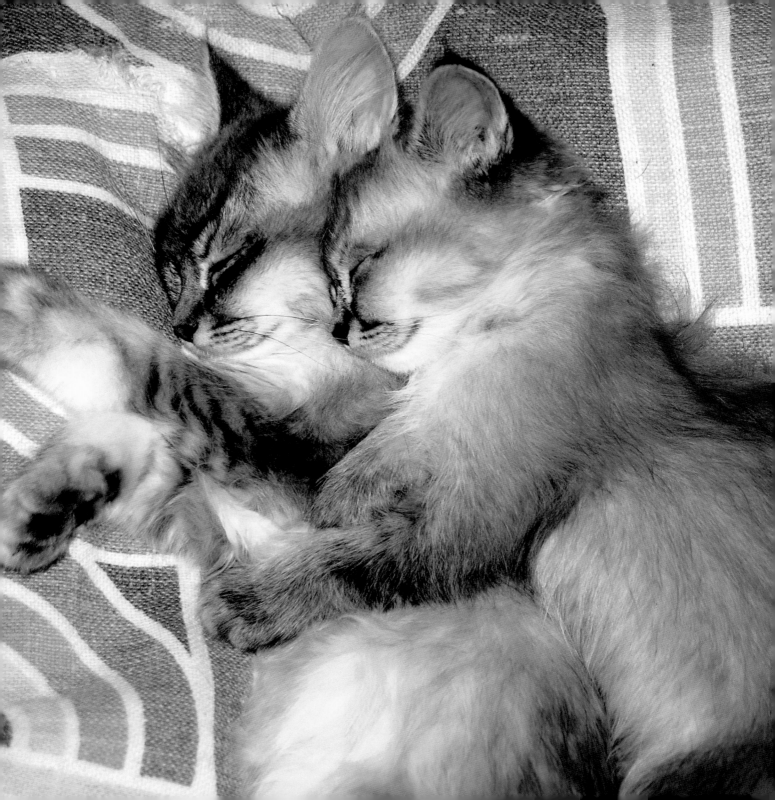

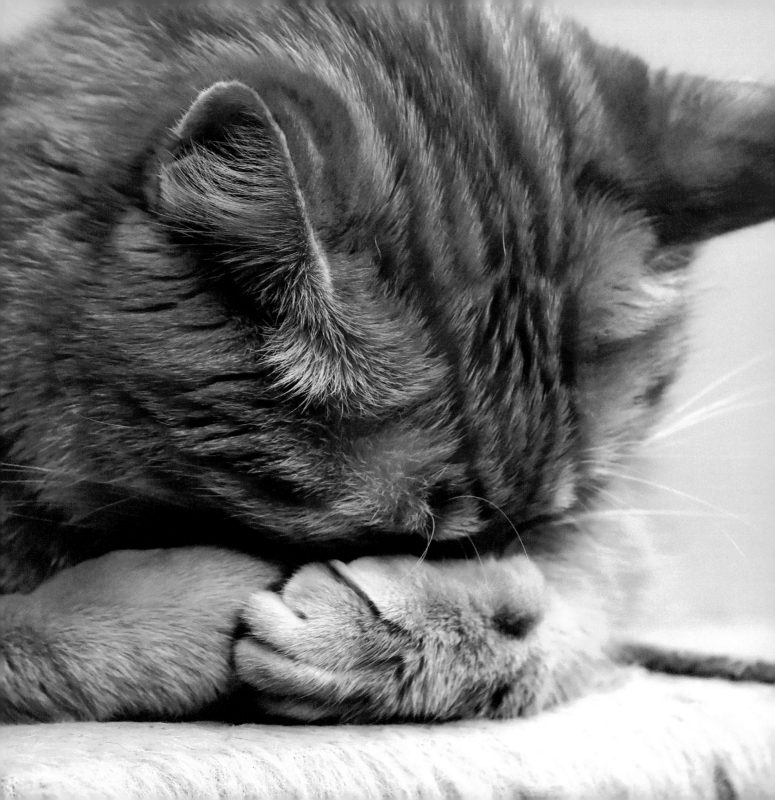

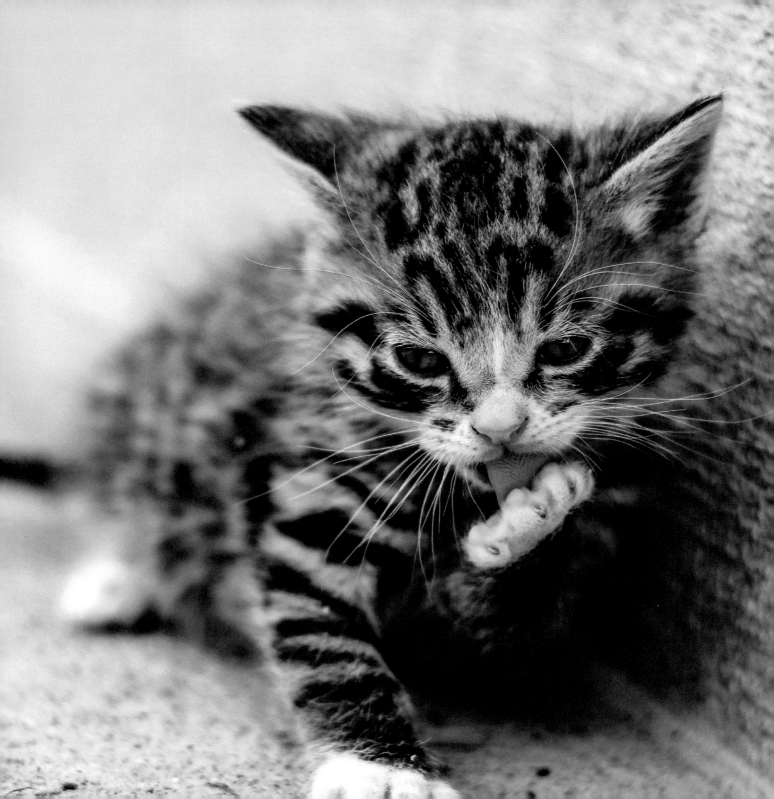

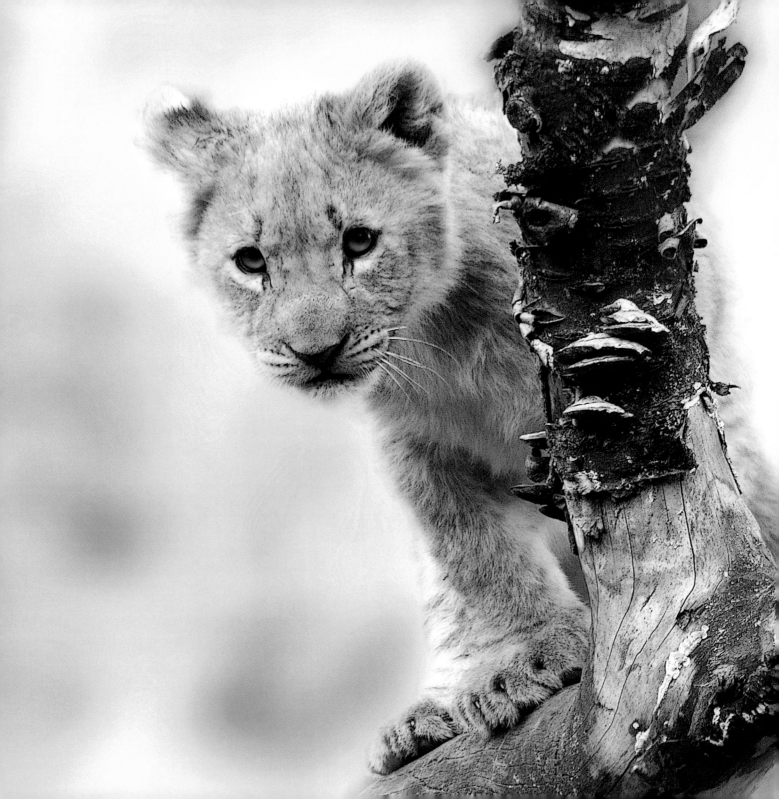

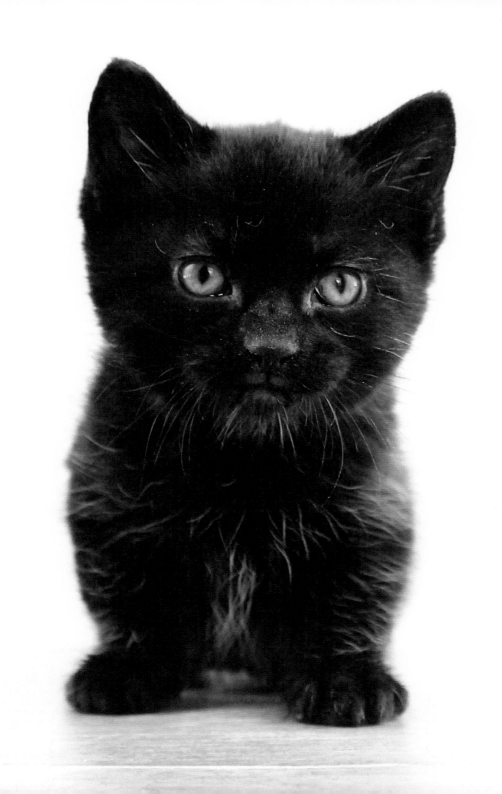

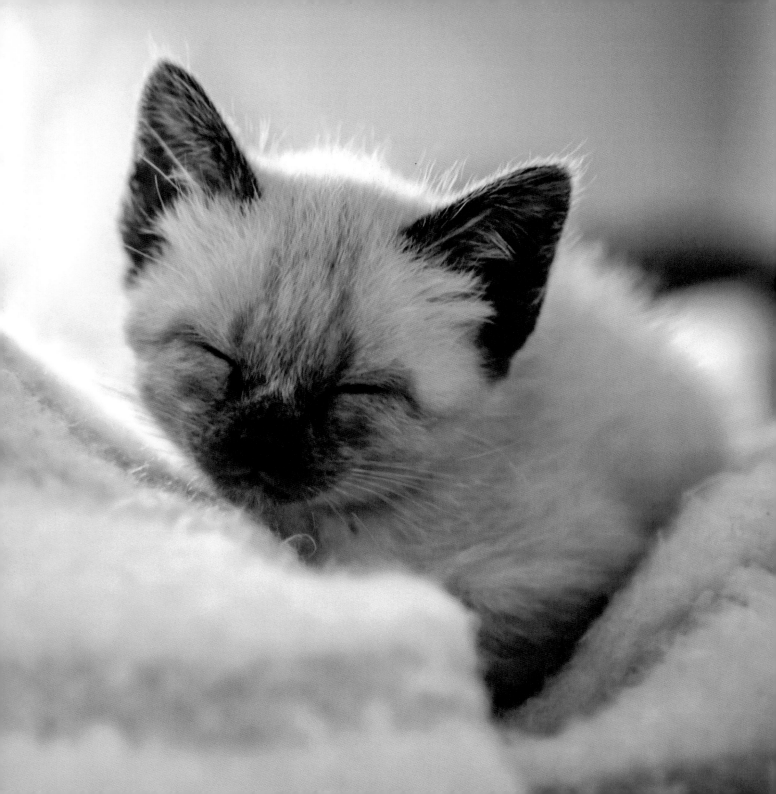

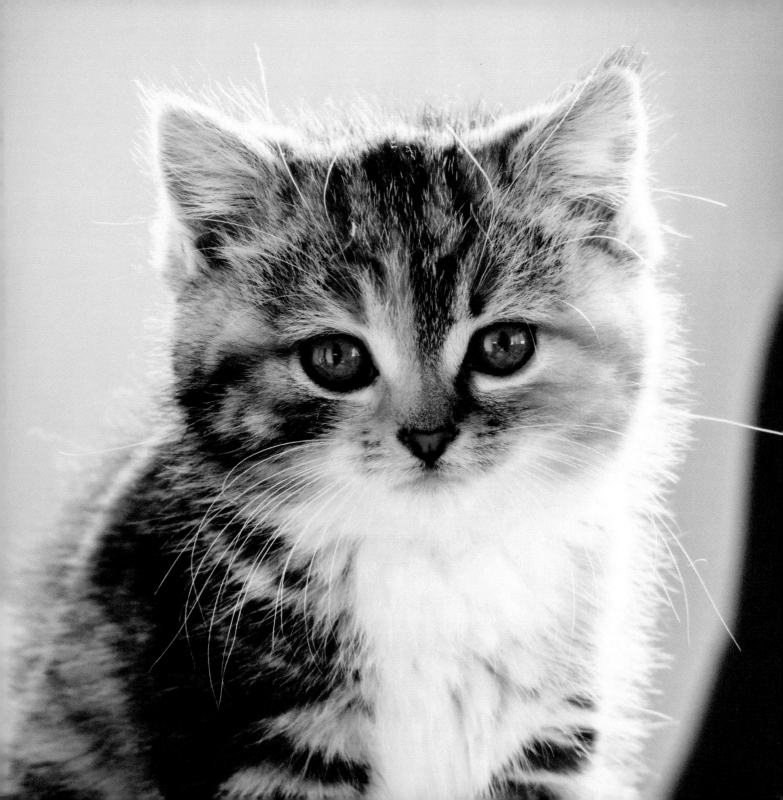

Please let me know what you thought of
my book by submitting a review on Amazon
or any other reader's website.

Books in this series:

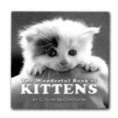 KITTENS

PUPPIES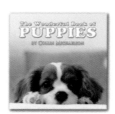

BABIES

BIRDS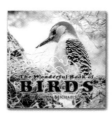

Printed in Great Britain
by Amazon